ESSENTIAL

MW01284615

Easy Ways to Supercharge Your Weight Loss Success with Essential Oils

Introduction

I want to thank you and congratulate you for downloading the book, *"Essential Oils for Weight Loss: Easy Ways to Supercharge Your Weight Loss Success with Essential Oils"* This book contains proven steps to help you reach your weight loss goals using the potent power of essential oils. Essential oils are natural oil extracts from fruits, plants, and seeds that when used in a variety of different ways, provide exceptional health benefits. The extraction of the oil is done primarily through steam distillation or cold pressing.

The use of essential oils dates back centuries to the time of the Ancient Egyptians around 3500 B.C. Since then we have learned even more about the amazing benefits of essential oils, especially as they relate to weight loss. By using a few simple oils either individually or in combination, you will see genuine and significant results. The beauty of most essential oils is their versatility. Many of the oils can be ingested, combined into a massage oil, or inhaled. The possibilities are almost endless. You can tailor the use of the oil to your preferences and use them in the ways that work best for you. I'm sure you will find the information useful and powerful in your weight loss journey.

Best of luck on your weight loss journey and beyond. Thanks again for downloading this book, I hope you enjoy it!

Chapter 1

Introduction to Essential Oils

Essential oil is by definition the oil extracted from a plant, seed, fruit or flower that contains the fragrance and essence of the plant from which it is extracted. But in reality, essential oils are so much more than that! They have been used for centuries dating back to ancient Egypt when they were used for religious ceremonies, medicines and cosmetics. Since then, the power of essential oils has been increasingly unfolding. We now know that they are extremely potent and can provide various health benefits including:

Stress and anxiety relief

Lower blood pressure

Disinfection

Cleaning

Antimicrobial

Antibacterial

Improved digestion

Allergy relief

Pain relief

Respiratory relief

Weight loss

The list goes on. There are literally hundreds of beneficial uses that essential oils can be used for depending on the particular type of oil. I think of essential oils as nature's pharmacy that provide the remedy that we need naturally, as long as we know where to look.

For those unfamiliar, there are a variety of ways in which essential oils can be administered. They are most commonly either used directly on the skin through massage, inhaled using a diffuser, or ingested. When being used in massage, the oils because of their potency, are usually mixed with a base oil or what's called a carrier oil before being applied to the skin. There are many different carrier oils such as grapeseed oil, sweet almond oil, olive oil, coconut oil and the list goes on. Please note that vegetable shortening, butter, margarine, and petroleum jelly should never be used as carrier oils. The carrier oil allows the effects of the oil to be experienced, while providing a protection to the skin and body.

 In some cases, you can apply the oils directly to the skin without mixing them with a carrier oil, but I would recommend consulting a licensed aromatherapist or essential oil specialist before doing so. There have been instances where undiluted direct contact with the skin has resulted in sensitization. Sensitization is basically similar to a skin allergy that results in a heavy rash or itchiness. More severe cases of sensitization can lead to respiratory problems or even anaphylactic shock. Once you become sensitized to an oil, you will likely continue to be sensitive to the oil, even if you use it in a diluted form with a carrier oil in the future. It's best to stay on the safe side.

Another way to use essential oils is to inhale the oils. There are many different methods to do this, including placing a drop or two on a cotton ball or tissue and inhaling it. This is a great method for when you're on the go. You can also do steam inhalation which is when you place 3-7 drops of essential oil into boiling water. Then cover your head with a towel and inhale. This is a great method to use when trying to clear up any sinus problems, or headaches. You can also use a diffuser and place a few drops of the essential oil in addition to water into the diffuser, and the diffuser will create a mist of the vapor mixed with the essential oil of your choice and spray it throughout the room. There are some really great diffusers available ranging in price from about $30 all the way up to $200+.

The third way to administer essential oils is through ingestion. You can ingest some oils and not others, it is best to do your own research about any oils you are planning to ingest before doing so. The oil must be processed by your liver, and as such you should take particular care not to overdo it when it comes to ingestion. Accumulation of large quantities of essential oils in the body can lead to liver and kidney damage. Keep in mind that in some cases, one drop of essential oil is equivalent to 75 cups of tea of that herb! If you would like to ingest your oils, use them sparingly, and mix them with honey before adding to your water or juice. We will touch on this again in more detail. This is not to scare you, but just to make you aware that you should treat essential oils with the same care as you do medicine.

Chapter 2

Essential Oils to Boost Weight Loss

In your weight loss journey, you will find several essential oils that will provide you with that added boost to push you towards reaching your goals. There are several essential oils that are excellent for boosting weight loss efforts. The beauty of essential oils is that they each have different properties and can produce different results. You can also try blending different oils together to harness and combine the different properties of the oils to achieve a variety of benefits.

Additionally, essential oils can be combined with aromatherapy in order to boost your weight loss. Aromatherapy stimulates parts of the brain that have positive effects on our emotional, physical and mental state. Breathing in fragrances stimulates the amygdala and the hippocampus which are the centers of human emotions and memory. Inhaling essential oils also stimulates brain receptors responsible for blood pressure, heart rate, attention span, stress and motivation.

Essential oils can provide an excellent supplemental boost to your weight loss plan. Many times, the struggle to lose weight has more to do with our psychological hurdles and burdens than it does with physical issues. Essential oils are great in this way because they can help you overcome some of the emotional or psychological blocks that have prevented successful weight loss in the past. For example, whether the issue is cravings for sweets, emotional eating, dieting fatigue, lack of motivation or slow metabolism, there is undoubtedly an essential oil or combination of oils that will alleviate the issue. Essential oils could be the missing ingredient that you need to finally achieve your weight loss goals.

Below you will find a list of essential oils and their properties and best uses for weight loss:

Grapefruit oil

Grapefruit oil is possibly the best essential oil to use to increase weight loss results. It suppresses appetite, boosts energy, reduces the appearance of cellulite, prevents bloating and dissolves fat. It contains nootkatone which is a natural chemical compound that stimulates a particular enzyme (AMPK specifically) which controls the body's energy levels and metabolism. AMPK hastens chemical reactions in the brain, liver and skeletal muscles. Research has shown that AMPK and nootkatone interact that results in improved endurance, reduced weight gain, decrease in body fat and increased physical performance.

It is also believed that limonene, a key hydrocarbon component found in grapefruit, creates lipolysis, a process where body fat is broken down and dissolved.

How to use it

Internally

Drink one glass of water with 1 or 2 drops of grapefruit essential oil. Be sure to buy high quality oil that is specifically made for internal use. It will help to get rid of toxins, lose excess fat, and weight management. You should aim to drink it in the morning so that you will benefit from its effects throughout the day.

Note: When ingesting essential oils, it's best to mix 1 or 2 drops with 1 tsp. of honey then add to warm water. This ensures safe absorption and processing by your body.

Massage

Add a few drops to a carrier oil such as extra virgin olive oil or unrefined virgin coconut oil. Massage it into into areas where fat accumulates thoroughly (about 30 minutes) and leave it on for a few hours before rinsing off.

Bath

Add 5 drops of grapefruit essential oil to you bath. Combine it with:

5 drops of ginger

5 drops of orange

5 drops of lemon

5 drops of sandalwood

Add a cup of apple cider vinegar

This combination will not only smell wonderful, but provides an excellent cellulite bath to aid with reducing the appearance of cellulite. Soak for approximately 30 minutes.

Caution: Always do a patch skin test first before applying any oil to the skin. You want to be sure that you are not allergic to any oil or oil combination before using them topically.

Lemon oil

This oil can be used to suppress appetite, increase energy and improve digestion. It aids the body in getting rid of toxins that would otherwise be stored in the fat cells. It has lots of great benefits aside from weight loss. When used as a mood enhancer, it is excellent at alleviating negative feelings. It also increases levels of norepinephrine a stress hormone which controls our fight or flight responses. In addition, norepinephrine increases oxygen in the brain for better brain function and improves blood flow and heart rate for optimal muscle functioning. In addition, lemon oil used in conjunction with grapefruit oil increases lipolysis.

Lemon oil is also good for getting rid of intestinal parasites, which contribute to weight gain.

How to use it:

Internally

Add 1 or 2 drops of lemon oil honey then to water in the morning before breakfast. This will help your body jumpstart your digestion and eliminate excess toxins.

Daily Massage

Add a few drops to a carrier oil of your choosing and massage into fat prone areas once per day. Helps eliminate toxins and waste stored in fat cells.

Peppermint oil

Since Peppermint is comprised of about 70% menthol, it has been traditionally used for hundreds of years to treat indigestion. It is an effective muscle relaxer, which helps relax the stomach muscles, reduce bloating and improve the flow of bile, which helps food pass through the body more quickly. Peppermint is also a natural appetite suppressant, and helps fight cravings.

How to use it:

Internally

Add 1 or 2 drops to honey then water before a meal to prevent overeating. Make sure to buy quality essential oils specifically for consumption (food grade).

Bath

Add 5-10 drops to your bathwater to invigorate your body and reduce food cravings.

It is said to be most effective in the mornings.

Inhalation

Add a couple of drops to a cotton ball and inhale it before a meal to act as an appetite suppressant. You can also put it into a zippered bag to take with you on the go.

Cinnamon Bark Oil

A great characteristic of cinnamon bark oil is that it helps you to feel full. It is best at preventing weight gain than actually losing weight, but it is a great complement to any other oils being used for weight loss. It helps the body break down sugars instead of storing them as fat. When the cells in the body cease to use insulin properly, this leads to a condition called insulin resistance. During insulin resistance the body mistakenly begins storing fat instead of burning it, which leads to weight gain or difficulty losing weight. This can lead to heightened blood sugar levels and insulin levels and result in pre-diabetes and possibly Type 2 diabetes. Cinnamon Bark has been shown to increase insulin sensitivity and thus help with blood glucose absorption.

Additionally, research has uncovered certain inflammatory cells while examining genetically obese people. Cinnamon extract has been shown to prevent the production of these cells, which may be a precursor to prevent weight gain.

How to use it:

Internally

Add 1 or 2 drops to water with a small amount of honey. Drink it before a meal or before going to bed to prevent cravings. Be sure to use high quality oil that is made for internal use.

Inhalation

Add a few drops to a cotton ball and inhale in order to prevent overeating and reduce appetite. You can place it into a Ziploc bag to take on the go.

Bergamot oil

The oil is derived from the Bergamot orange, a sour orange that is inedible, but whose essence and oils provide many health benefits. Bergamot oranges are widely grown in Italy, where more than 80% of the fruit is produced. Bergamot peel is also used in fragrance production, and is used as a component of Earl Grey tea.

The beauty of Bergamot is that it helps calm the nerves and additionally acts as a mood lifter and antidepressant by stimulating the endocrine system. Many times we tend to eat when we are stressed or emotionally taxed. The smell of Bergamot can help you relax, lift your spirits and keep you from eating when you are not truly hungry. Bergamot also is full of polyphenols, which help your body to burn fats and sugars. Bergamot is usually not ingested.

How to use it:

Inhalation

Place a few drops to a cloth and inhale it when you are feeling tempted to grab food when you're not actually hungry.

Foot & Neck Rub

Add a few drops of the oil to a carrier oil such as olive or coconut oil. Gently massage your neck and feet to relieve stress and relax. Additionally, you can use Bergamot to in conjunction with Sandalwood oil to de-stress and overcome negative feelings.

Please be aware that Bergamot is particularly photosensitive, meaning that you should avoid exposing areas treated with Bergamot to direct sunlight for up to 3 days after topical application.

Orange oil

The oil can be used to reduce depression, as well as improve endocrine and immune system functioning. It has great anti - inflammatory properties and when used internally. It can help with gas and bloating, indigestion, fever, infections as well as assist with weight loss. It is also a diuretic and it promotes urination which helps rid the body of toxins such as bile, uric acid, extra salt, pollutants and excess water.

It also comprised of 85%-95% limonene, which similar to grapefruit oil, helps break down and dissolve fat.

How to use it:

Internally

Add a drop or two to your water or meal. Once again, be sure that the oil is specifically for internal use (food grade).

Massage

Add a few drops to the carrier oil of your choice and massage into the skin such as jojoba, sweet almond or avocado oil.

Inhalation

A few drops of the oil can be added to a cotton ball or cloth and inhaled. You can also add a few drops to a warm bath.

Caution: Orange oil as well as many of the other citrus oils such as lemon, bergamot, and grapefruit, among others can cause photo toxicity. What this means is that if you apply the oil directly to skin and then immediately expose the skin to natural sunlight or sunbed radiation, it may cause severe burns or possible cancers. You will need to wait at least 12 hours after topical application before exposing to natural or sunbed radiation. So please be aware of this when using.

Sandalwood oil

Mainly known for its exotic and intoxicating scent, it has been used for centuries in various applications. It works to balance the emotions as well as the immune system. It will provide you with an overall sense of well-being which can be a great help if trying to overcome emotional eating. It has a high concentration of sesquiterpenes which is a naturally occurring chemical compound found in many essential oils that promotes health and wellness, particularly as it relates to brain function. It is one of the few oils that is known to flow between the blood brain barrier, which is necessary in order to fight brain diseases.

It also helps the digestive system by soothing upset stomachs, relieving gas, heartburn and diarrhea, and generally calming the whole digestive system.

How to use it:

Internally

Dilute by adding a couple of drops into a glass of water or juice.

Inhalation

Fill a large bowl or basin with steaming hot water and add a few drops of oil and place head over the steaming bowl and breathe in. It is also helpful to cover head with a towel to keep the vapor from escaping.

Fennel Seed Oil

Fennel seed oil has various positive benefits on weight loss including acting as a metabolic enhancer and appetite suppressant. By increasing the metabolic rate, helps the body burn calories faster and accelerates weight loss. Fennel also helps break up fat deposits in the bloodstream to be used as energy. A German study found that dieters who supplemented their diets with fennel seed ate less.

Fennel also contains melatonin, which is a natural hormone that regulates sleep cycles, and also helps control weight gain. It also promotes urination and thus helps the body flush out toxins and get rid of water weight and bloating.

How to use it:

Internally

You can add a couple of drops to water or other beverages. In addition, you can make a fennel seed water, which uses the full fennel seed steeped in hot water or immersed in cool water overnight. (see recipe below)

Overnight steeping method

- 1 liter/ 4 cups of drinking water

- 2 tablespoons of raw fennel seeds

In this method, all you have to do is to get a glass jar, pour in 2 tablespoons of fennel seeds and fill it up with 1 liter of water. Then, cover it with a lid and you can forget about it until the next morning. At first the seeds will be floating at the top, but by morning the seeds will be engorged with water and will have sunk to the bottom.

It is advisable to start out drinking one cup of fennel water during the day, to see if you have any allergic or other adverse reactions to it. Once you've tested it and are fine, feel free to drink the full liter throughout the day. Caution: fennel and fennel water should not be consumed or used by pregnant or nursing women.

Chapter 3

How to integrate essential oils into your weight loss plan

Using essential oils to help you reach your weight loss goals is a great decision. The natural compounds and components found in the oils are the perfect supplement to help you avoid cravings, suppress appetite, and boost your metabolism. You will need a plan in addition to the oils in order to be successful however. You can't run around eating double cheeseburgers and fries every day without exercising and expect to lose weight from the oils alone. They are wonderful tools to use, but you should also follow an eating and exercise plan to stay on track as well.

So here are some helpful tips that you can use to work towards your weight loss goal. This is a six week weight loss plan provided by health.com

1. *Eat protein and fruit and/or vegetables at every meal*

To help give your body all of the amino acids it needs in order to support muscle building and tone, you need to include a protein and a fruit or veggie at each meal. You can have 3 to 4 ounces of chicken or turkey, lean beef (sirloin, tenderloin or roasts are good options), or seafood, whether fresh, frozen or canned. Just be aware that you shouldn't have more than 6 oz. per week of albacore tuna because it contains higher levels of mercury than other types of tuna.

Getting a good amount of protein with each meal will keep you full and hopefully prevent you from reaching for bad snacks.

2. *Eat fruit and nuts*

When it is time for a snack, eating unsalted nuts or seeds and fruit twice a day is a good choice. Nuts are high in heart healthy fats, protein, fiber and antioxidants. Opt for lower calorie nuts such as almonds or cashews rather than higher calorie nuts like brazil or macadamia nuts.

3. *Avoid dairy, soy & grains*

For the first half of your eating plan, say three or four weeks, try to stay away from dairy, soy or grain products. The reason is because they can cause food sensitivities to flare up, resulting in bloating, low energy and unhealthy skin. Food sensitivities "can cause a low grade inflammation in every part of your body from your heart to your bones to your skin." Says diet creator Christine Lydon, MD.

Starting around the fourth week, you can start adding about 100 calories per meal of dairy or soy products. After week 5 you can have up to 100 calories per meal of whole grain sourced foods such as oatmeal, ½ cup of whole grain pasta, a slice of whole grain bread, 1/3 cup of brown rice, potatoes or sweet potatoes. If you notice bloating or sluggishness, then cut back as before.

4. *Cut out the processed foods*

It's best to leave the chips, cookies and processed food for the entire 6 week plan, and then eat them in moderation only afterwards. The reason is because these foods lead to inflammation and speed up the aging process.

5. *Drink when you eat*

You should drink between 10 to 12 oz. of fluids each time you have a meal or snack. You should aim for water, sparkling water, unsweetened green tea. Stay away from soda, even diet soda which research shows is processed similar to other sugary snacks and may increase cravings for sweets. You can flavor your drinks with lemon, lime and berry juice. You can also have up to two black coffees or teas.

6. *Take your vitamins*

Take a daily multi vitamin during this time. In addition, you may want to try using myrrh essential oil, wintergreen or oregano oil mixed with a carrier oil and rubbed into sore or inflamed areas. Be sure your multivitamin contains at least 5 micrograms of vitamin D to help with the absorption of calcium.

Workout plan

This workout plan was designed to be done in 20 minutes five times per week for three weeks. Don't rest in between exercises, but continue the entire way through.

Step ups
Body parts worked: quads, glutes, hamstrings

Step onto a low bench or platform with right foot, then left foot. Step down with right foot, then left foot. Do 20 reps, then repeat with left foot.

Push ups
Body parts worked: shoulders, chest, triceps

Place your hands shoulder width apart on the floor then walk your feet back until they are straight and your body is parallel to the floor. Slowly bend arms and lower chest towards the floor. When elbows form a 90 degree angle, push back up to starting position. Do 30 reps.

Lunge curls
Body parts worked: glutes, hamstrings, quads

While holding a 5-8 pound dumbbell in each hand, start with feet together and arms at both sides. Step forward with your left foot and lower your right knee towards the floor. Left leg should form a 90 degree angle. Don't let your knee go past your ankle. At the same time, curl weights towards your shoulders and chest. Return to the starting position and repeat with right foot. Do 20 reps per leg.

Squeeze crunches

Body parts worked: hamstrings, glutes, abs

Lie on your back with arms near ears and elbows pointing outward. Place a small pillow behind your knees, squeeze and pull your knees towards your chest. Continue to squeeze the pillow as you move your shoulder blades off of the floor, moving your nose towards your knees. Hold for a moment, then return to starting position. Do 30 reps.

Squat presses
Body parts worked: glutes, hamstrings, quads, shoulders, core

Holding 3- to 5-pound dumbbells beside shoulders, stand with feet twice shoulder-width apart. Keep back straight as you squat until thighs are almost parallel to the floor; push through heels and press weights up as you return to standing. Do 30 reps.

Rows
Body parts worked: biceps, back

Holding 5- to 8-pound dumbbells by your sides, stand with feet shoulder-width apart and back about a foot from the wall. Press butt against the wall for support, then bend at the knees and waist so torso and thighs form a right angle. Keeping head up and back straight, draw elbows straight back and up, bringing weights up to touch torso. Pause, then lower weights. Do 30 reps.

Squat rises
Body parts worked: quads, glutes, hamstrings, shoulders

Stand with feet shoulder-width apart, holding 3- to 5-pound dumbbells by your sides. Keeping back straight, squat until thighs are nearly parallel to the floor, then push off balls of feet to rise back to standing as you raise dumbbells out to sides until parallel with shoulders. Return to starting position. Do 30 reps.

Squeeze side crunches
Body parts worked: hamstrings, abs

Lie on back with hands by ears and elbows pointing out. Place a small pillow behind knees, squeeze, and bring knees toward chest. Continue to squeeze the pillow as you move left elbow toward right knee, lifting left shoulder blade. Hold for a beat, then lower back down. Repeat on opposite side. Do 15 reps per side.

Door squats

Body parts worked: glutes, quads

Stand with feet shoulder-width apart, one on either side of front edge of an open door. Grasp a towel looped around both doorknobs, extend arms, and lean back. Keep back straight. Bend knees and lower butt toward floor. Pause, tighten butt muscles and rise back up. When legs straighten, thrust pelvis forward, squeezing butt muscles again. Do 30 reps.

Bench dips

Body parts worked: triceps, shoulders, chest

Sit on bench edge with hands on either side of butt. Slide butt off and extend legs until straight. Keeping torso upright, bend elbows as you lower butt toward floor. When upper arms are nearly parallel to floor, push back up to starting position. Do 20 reps.

Chapter 4

Essential oils for cellulite

Ah the dreaded cellulite. It is one of the most hated occurrences that (mainly women) have to deal with. Cellulite is a result mainly of aging and that occurs as a result of the loss of elasticity in the body's tissues. It can also be caused by poor circulation, fluid retention, heredity, and hormones such as estrogen and progesterone. It is extremely unflattering to look at, and is usually visible on the legs and upper thighs. All is not lost though, essential oils can aid in melting this unsightly fat away. Below you will find some tips on how to utilize essential oils to get rid of cellulite once and for all.

Cypress essential oil

Is a strong oil that boosts the body's circulatory functions and helps prevent fluid retention from building up in the body. It also helps with removal of toxins from the body. Controlling all these harmful types of buildups also leads to elimination of bad body fats and cellulite.

To use:

Mix a few drops with a carrier oil of your choice and massage into areas that have cellulite twice per day. You may also choose to use a dry soft bristled shower body brush to massage the oil into problem areas.

Some carrier oils that are commonly used in the fight against cellulite are:

Avocado oil, coconut oil, jojoba oil, walnut oil and sweet almond oil.

Rosemary oil

It is best known for its use in cooking and culinary creations, but it also provides wonderful benefits in fighting cellulite and fat deposits. The oil is extracted from the evergreen plant the rosemary. It is great for improving circulation. It has a warming effect on the body which helps blood circulate throughout. It is also a great antioxidant and diuretic. It helps remove toxins from the body and reduce cellulite simultaneously.

To use:

Mix with a carrier oil or lotion of your choice such as almond oil or wheat germ oil.

Grapefruit oil

Among its other great properties, grapefruit oil is great for lowering water retention and preventing lymph accumulation (lymphedema or fluid accumulation in the tissues) which often results in cellulite. It contains bromelain an anti-inflammatory enzyme that breaks down cellulite. It has the added benefit of clearing up acne and oily skin problems.

To use:

Add a few drops to carrier oil and massage into affected areas daily for best results.

Lemon oil

Is a stimulant to the circulatory system and even improves microcirculation. It is found to be successful at treating varicose veins as well by improving circulation and relieving pressure on the veins (when combined with Cypress oil in a 1 to 1 ratio).

To use:

Add a few drops to a carrier oil and massage into problem areas.

Geranium oil

Is a great hormonal balancer, and is wonderful at getting rid of cellulite and stretch marks. It does its magic by helping with fluid retention. It also assists with detoxification of the body by acting as a diuretic.

To use:

Add a few drops to the carrier oil of your choosing and massage into fat prone areas.

Spearmint Oil

Spearmint is a potent antibacterial and anti-inflammatory oil. It also helps regulate the body's absorption of fat. When used in conjunction with grapefruit oil, its powers are magnified. It will also make you feel great, creating a sense of balance and overall well-being.

To use:

Add a few drops to the carrier oil of your choice and massage into problem areas. You may choose to add grapefruit oil to a blend, as the two oils enhance each other.

Cellulite Essential Oil Blend Recipes

These recipes will get you started on your way to finally being free of that pesky cellulite. Feel free to try a few of these to see which ones work best, or create your own blend. Just remember to add no more than 5-6 drops of each essential oil to every 10 ml of carrier oil. At maximum for a 100 ml bottle for example, you should use no more than 60 drops of essential oil.

Classic Cellulite Blend

Rosemary 10 drops

Geranium 10 drops

Juniper 20 drops

Spearmint 10 drops and grapefruit 10 drops.

Mix into 100mls of organic base oil.

Directions:

Massage into skin as needed, twice per day for best results. When this remedy is finished, change the rosemary, geranium and grapefruit for eucalyptus, black pepper and lavender. It is good to alternate the remedy as it gives your body an extra boost. When this bottle is empty, return to the original formula.

Grapefruit Cellulite Cream

30 drops grapefruit essential oil

1 cup coconut oil

Glass jar

Directions:

Mix grapefruit oil and coconut oil together

Rub on cellulite areas for a few minutes daily.

Store in container when not in use. Citrus oils are very acidic and may eat away at plastic containers.

Grapefruit cellulite oil

Ingredients

> ½ cup olive oil (can also use almond, jojoba or even coffee infused oil)
>
> 15 drops grapefruit essential oil
>
> 15 drops juniper essential oil
>
> 5 drops rosemary essential oil

Directions:

Combine all oils in a glass jar and stir.

Apply a small amount of oil to skin.

During first four weeks, massage oil into skin using a circular motion twice a day.

For ongoing use, apply daily.

Homemade Cellulite Cream

All you need to make this badass homemade cellulite cream is a few essential oils and a base:

- 3/4 cup Coconut Oil

- 2 tablespoons shaved Beeswax

- 3 tablespoons Witch Hazel

- 10 drops Juniper oil

- 10 drops Rosemary oil

- 30 drops Grapefruit oil

- 30 drops Cypress oil

Directions:

Step 1 – Start by mixing together all of your essential oils and your witch hazel. Stir until evenly blended.

Step 2 – Over low heat, melt your beeswax then add in your coconut oil, if it is not liquid yet.

Step 3 – Once your beeswax and coconut oil is in liquid form, add it to your essential oil bowl and blend.

Step 4 – Pour contents into an easily sealable jar and store in a cool, dry place.

Anti-cellulite lotion

Ingredients:

125 ml Unscented natural lotion base

8 drops of Lavender, juniper and geranium essential oils

Then add double of the quantity above which is 16 drops of each Cypress and Lemon Essential Oil

Plus 20 ml Witch Hazel

Directions:

Mix all the ingredients into a cup until the texture is uniform. The mixture may then be placed in a clean bottle. It is advised that this blend be applied after shower in the morning. The application is procedurally done by circular-upward motion until the applied amount is absorbed by the skin.

Grapefruit Cellulite Scrub

½ cup sugar

½ cup coffee grounds (fresh or used)

½ cup oil (pick your favorite - almond, olive, coconut, etc.)

15-20 drops grapefruit essential oil

Directions:

Combine ingredients in a bowl, stirring together to thoroughly mix and create a thick paste.

Add more oil or sugar to get desired consistency.

Store in a lidded container. Will last several months unless water it introduced.

To use, apply to skin and scrub in circular motions over areas with cellulite.

General words of caution:

If you are new to using essential oils, I would recommend consulting a licensed aromatherapist before use. Essential oils while natural, have very powerful properties that you should know well prior to use. All oils are not the same. Do your research on each oil, use your best judgement, and if in doubt be conservative and start with small quantities. Knowing your body, your own sensitivities and reactions is key. Essential oils can be a great source of healing and enhance your health and well-being, just be sure to use them properly and wisely.

Chapter 5

Where to buy essential oils?

One thing is for sure, not all essential oils are created equal. More specifically, not all essential oil companies create the same quality oils. It is key that you only purchase the highest quality oils and make sure that the oils you are using are appropriate for the method you are using (ie: if you are taking oil internally, you want to be sure that it is food grade). Some companies dilute their "100% pure" essential oils with other carrier or base oils and you really have no idea what you are actually getting. It's best to do your own research as to which brand to purchase from, but I have a few companies that I have used that you may want to check out. I recommend that you conduct your own research on the best suppliers to buy your oils from.

Mountain Rose Herbs- They are all organic and pesticide free. They are a great company with lovely smelling oils for reasonable prices. They source their oils only from distillers that they know and trust.

Plant Therapy- They promote safe practices of essential oil use, have fair prices for their high quality oils, and even have a child friendly line of oils.

Native American Nutritionals- Very nice smelling oils that are said to be some of the finest quality oils on the market. The company's owner ensures that the oils are harvested from their native regions where he feels the oils will have the best plant essence.

Aura Cacia- Nice smelling oils that are said to have excellent quality chemistry.

Some other factors that you may want to take into consideration when choosing an essential oil supplier can be found below:

Is the company eco-friendly?

This is because many companies harvest plants that are endangered or have company practices that aren't sustainable or eco-friendly.

Are they a smaller company versus a larger corporation?

A smaller company may have (not always) tighter controls over their product or be more conscious of the way in which their oils are produced.

Does the company have relationships with their distillers (if possible)?

Can the company provide material safety data sheets (MSDS) if necessary?

These are sheets that tell you how to handle the oil safely and what to do in case of emergency.

Are they a supplier with an overall good reputation in the industry?

Any major scandals or lots of customer complaints is probably a red flag.

Are they owned by an aromatherapy practitioner or essential oil specialist?

Not necessary, but usually an indication of quality products.

Conclusion

Thank you again for downloading this book!

I hope this book was able to help you learn about essential oils and their amazing properties in relation to weight loss. Essential oils are a great tool to use in reaching your weight loss goals, and when used properly and in conjunction with a eating and exercise plan will likely give your fabulous results. I

hope you have learned that you don't need to spend a fortune

on expensive commercial weight loss pills or cellulite creams in order to see great results. The best part is that essential oils are natural, and you can create your own wonderful blends that suit your needs and preferences. I hope you are excited about your journey and I wish you nothing but the best in this and all your endeavors.

All the best,

Isla

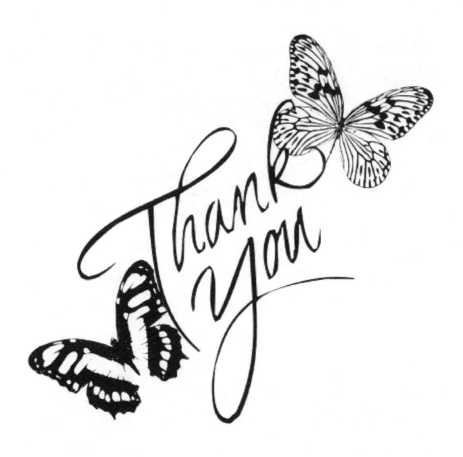

Finally, if you enjoyed this book, then I'd like to ask you for a favor, would you be kind enough to leave a review for this book on Amazon? It'd be greatly appreciated!

Thank you and good luck!

Preview Of 'Aromatherapy and Essential Oils for Beginners: The Ultimate Guide to Essential Oils for Health, Beauty & Home'

Chapter 1-

What exactly are Aromatherapy & Essential Oils?

Aromatherapy is simple at its core. It is the practice of using oils extracted from nuts, seeds, flowers, leaves, fruits, and twigs for special restorative purposes. These oils called essential oils, work in harmony with the body to produce powerful beneficial effects and have the ability to improve a person's well -being both physically and mentally.

It has long been used to treat and relieve a variety of conditions including burns, infections, depression and high blood pressure among others. In addition, essential oils are known to have antibacterial properties when applied to the skin. One study discovered that when essential oils were inhaled, markers from the fragrance could be found in the blood, showing that aromatherapy was acting similar to a drug. Because of their special properties, the effects that the oils produce are difficult to replicate, and the benefits are most profoundly seen when using the essential oils.

The use of essential oils goes back thousands of years and is attributed to the Egyptians who used them for medicines, cosmetics and in their religious practices. Aromatic resins were also used in parts of the embalming process.

In addition to oils, aromatherapy uses other natural ingredients like vegetable oils, jojoba (a liquid wax), herbs, sea salts, clays and muds to achieve similar beneficial results. Aromatherapists may place the oils on the skin during a massage, or alternatively, use the oils as sprays or in diffusers to freshen their homes. There are various ways that the oils can be used:

Indirect inhalation-person inhales the oils using a diffuser or by placing drops in a container in the room.

Direct inhalation –person inhales the oils using an inhaler with drops floating on top of hot water. (ie: to treat a headache)

Massage- essential oils are massaged into the skin.

Mixing- essential oils are mixed into lotions, creams or bath salts.

The fragrance of the essential oil stimulates the nerves of the nose. The nerves send impulses to the brain that control memory and emotion. The effect of each oil is different, but generally, the oil will either be calming or stimulating.

There have also been many studies done to measure the effect of aromatherapy in cancer patients. The results show that aromatherapy may improve quality of life in patients with cancer. Some patients receiving aromatherapy have reported improvement in symptoms such as nausea or pain, and have lower blood pressure pulse, and respiratory rates. Studies of aromatherapy massage have had mixed results, with some studies reporting improvement in mood, anxiety, pain, and constipation and other studies reporting no effect. *

In 1998 a UK study looked at the effects of aromatherapy in 58 cancer patients. Most of these patients were women with breast cancer who said that they would like aromatherapy to help them with feelings of stress, anxiety, depression and fear. Each patient had 6 aromatherapy treatments during the study. At the end of these treatments all the patients showed a significant improvement in their feelings of anxiety, depression and stress.**

*cancer.org

**cancerresearchuk.org

Chapter 2

Starting to use essential oils

Getting treatment from an aromatherapist

When they are being massaged into the skin, essential oils are usually blended with another oil called a carrier oil. It is usually a vegetable oil and is called a carrier oil because of its ability to carry oil to the skin. Essential oils are especially concentrated and if used directly on the skin could cause damage. This is why the carrier oil is needed.

The most common types of carrier oils are:

Olive oil

Jojoba oil

Almond oil

Grapeseed oil

Avocado oil

Coconut oil

When you have your first aromatherapy massage, the aromatherapist will probably ask you about lifestyle and health. If you have a serious or complicated medical condition, they may ask to speak with your primary doctor to make sure it's medically advisable for you to receive aromatherapy treatment. The aromatherapist will choose the oils that they know will help your specific condition and help manage your symptoms the best. They will massage the oils gently into your skin. The session will normally last between an hour and an hour and a half. They may play relaxing music during the session as well. It is usually a very calming and relaxing experience.

Using essential oils at home

When you are at home and want to make your own aromatherapy treatment, it is relatively easy to do so. You can add essential oils to water and use an oil burner to inhale them. Adding the essential oils to hot or boiling water is a great method for getting started.

Check Out My Other Books

Below you'll find some of my other popular books that are popular on Amazon and Kindle as well. Simply click on the links below to check them out. Alternatively, you can visit my author page on Amazon to see other work done by me.

Simply Bliss: Easy Ways to Organize and De-Stress Your Life Forever

Meditation for Beginners: How to Meditate to Decrease Stress & Vastly Improve Health and Happiness

Positive Affirmations: Positive Affirmations for Health & Wealth That Will Transform Your Life Forever